Distribution, publication, and copying in any form are prohibited and subject to damages.

TEN HYPNOSES

Distribution, publication, and copying in any form are prohibited and subject to damages.

Copying, publishing, and sharing with third parties are only permitted with the written consent of the author. Please observe the notes on copyright and usage.

Distribution, publication, and copying in any form are prohibited and subject to damages.

Ingo Michael Simon

TEN HYPNOSES

20
SOCIAL PHOBIA AND FEAR OF CONTACT

Copying, publishing, and sharing with third parties are only permitted with the written consent of the author. Please observe the notes on copyright and usage.

Distribution, publication, and copying in any form are prohibited and subject to damages.

© 2024 Ingo Michael Simon
All rights reserved.
Independently published
www.ingosimon.com

Important Notes for Urgent Attention:
The contents of this book are based on the practical experiences of the author with hypnosis applications and psychotherapy in a trance state. Although the author has strived for the utmost care, errors or misunderstandings in the presentation cannot be completely excluded. Therapeutic work with people and the application of hypnosis are solely the responsibility of the hypnotist. It cannot be ruled out that parts of this book may be misunderstood or that the application of a presented procedure may cause an undesirable reaction in the client. The author also assumes no co-responsibility if work with a client is carried out with reference to the statements in this book.

The Author:
Ingo Michael Simon studied psychology and education and is a hypnotherapist with practices in southwestern Germany and Switzerland. With the help of hypnosis-supported psychotherapy, he primarily treats people with persistent psychological conditions. His practice focuses on anxiety disorders, pathological compulsions, and psychosomatic illnesses. His therapeutic offerings mainly include classical and modern hypnosis applications and the dreamland therapy he developed himself.

Copying, publishing, and sharing with third parties are only permitted with the written consent of the author. Please observe the notes on copyright and usage.

Notes on Copyright and Usage

Copying, publishing, and sharing with third parties is prohibited and only permitted with the written consent of the author. Please observe the following copyright and usage guidelines.

This work has been carefully crafted and created to the best of the author's knowledge and personal experience. It comprises text templates and application guidelines for professional hypnosis sessions. The author is a licensed psychotherapist with extensive experience in psychotherapy, coaching, and personal training using hypnotic techniques and methods. Nevertheless, the author and the publisher assume no liability for the accuracy of information, instructions, and advice, nor for any typographical errors. The author and publisher accept no responsibility or liability for the application of these texts and recommendations with clients or patients, nor for any potential consequences or unexpected reactions. It is expressly noted that the application of therapeutic and advisory techniques and formulations lies solely and entirely within the responsibility of the practitioner. This also applies to adherence to the boundaries of legally regulated medical and therapeutic practices. The fact that a book containing action proposals is freely available for sale does not imply that its application with clients or patients is permitted for everyone.

Distribution, publication, and copying in any form are prohibited and subject to damages.

Copying, publishing, and sharing with third parties are only permitted with the written consent of the author. Please observe the notes on copyright and usage.

Distribution, publication, and copying in any form are prohibited and subject to damages.

Table of Contents

Introduction 9

#1 11

#2 17

#3 23

#4 29

#5 35

#6 40

#7 45

#8 50

#9 55

#10 60

Overview of All Titles in the Series "Ten Hypnoses" 65

Copying, publishing, and sharing with third parties are only permitted with the written consent of the author. Please observe the notes on copyright and usage.

Distribution, publication, and copying in any form are prohibited and subject to damages.

Copying, publishing, and sharing with third parties are only permitted with the written consent of the author. Please observe the notes on copyright and usage.

Introduction

The series "Ten Hypnoses" is very well known in Germany, Austria, and Switzerland as a collection of texts for therapeutic work and is used by numerous psychotherapeutic practices, doctors, therapists, coaches, and other helping professionals. I am pleased to now be able to offer these texts in other countries as well.

Most therapists have their own methods for inducing and deepening trance as well as for exiting trance. Therefore, I have focused on the main part of the hypnosis. The texts in this book can be integrated as the main part into any hypnosis process.

The texts in this collection use various hypnosis techniques. I will not explain these in detail, as I assume that users have the appropriate training. It is also not necessary to understand the exact structure or functioning of the different parts. The texts can simply be read aloud, and they will have their effect.

Decide for yourself which text best suits your client or patient at any given time. You can also combine passages from different texts. It is not about using all ten hypnoses in sequence. It is a selection of possibilities.

I want to emphasize that books cannot replace therapy. Psychotherapy or other therapeutic treatments involve much more. A careful diagnosis is the necessary basis for deciding on the use of methods, including whether hypnosis or one of my texts should be used. Even in this case, preparatory discussions, follow-up discussions during the session, and of course, a therapeutic concept for the sequence of sessions and the content approaches are essential parts of therapy. This cannot and should not be achieved with a collection of texts.

In any case, I wish you much success in your work and I am pleased if my text templates can contribute in a small way.

Ingo Michael Simon

#1

You have made an important decision ... ... You have decided to be brave and confident again from now on ... ... You have a clear goal in mind and pursue it with all your strength ... ... You know what you want ... ... You want to be strong and courageous when interacting with other people ... ... looking the people around you straight in the eye and feeling good about it ... ... That is your goal ... ... and you can achieve this goal today ... ... faster than you think ... ... The solution to your fear lies deep within you ... ... Freed from fear, it will be easy to meet others ... ... you can experience it calmly and quietly ... ... here and now in your imagination and tomorrow in your waking reality ... ... and then every day because you have decided it internally ... ... It's admirable how well you manage to fully enter into this inner attitude ... ... this attitude that outwardly shows that you are confident and calm ... ... You start by gathering your strength ... ... All the energy in your body flows into your legs ... ... your legs provide a firm stand ... ... You stand firmly on the outside and you feel the stability and strength growing within you ... ... It's truly amazing how important strong legs are for a good and strong feeling ... ... and it's really astonishing how quickly your legs have changed their posture ... ... maybe you already feel it yourself ... ... or in a few moments you will clearly feel that your legs have become strong ... ... strong like you ... ... strong like you ... ...

Then you stand beside yourself and observe your body ... ... You see yourself standing on both legs ... ... upright and strong ... ... stable and self-assured ... ... supported by your own strength ... ... Stable and unshakeable, you stand on both legs ... ... Your stance becomes firmer ... ... Nothing could shake you ... ... This feeling grows stronger and stronger ... ... this feeling that gives you support and security ... ... Self-confidence within you ... ... Self-confidence that has always been within you ... ... always within you ... ... and it is amazing how your body implements this for you, showing you your own strength and letting you feel your own power ... ... Then you feel the strength in your arms as well ... ... They are strong and powerful ... ... much stronger than you may have thought ... ... because your arms also show you that this very power lies within you … … This strength that impresses others … … this proud posture that impresses other people more than you thought … … They see you very differently than you have seen yourself until now … … For other people, you are much bigger and stronger than you have seen yourself … … because you are actually bigger and stronger … … much bigger and much stronger … … and today you succeed more than ever in feeling this size and strength as well … … Your shoulders are also stable and strong … … They hold your body in a proud position … … just like that … … just like that … … You breathe freely in and out … … just like now … … You take a deep breath and feel your own strength more and more … … Strength in your legs … … Strength in your arms … … Strength in your shoulders … … You stand as secure as a tree … … You feel your own strength growing stronger and stronger … … Your head is held high and stable … … Your gaze is fixed straight ahead … … Your face relaxes and you feel good … … You take a deep breath and feel good in this strength … … People pass by you … … You observe them with your head held high and a firm gaze … … They hurry past you … … But you stand firm and stable … … You feel your strength … … You let all these people pass by you ... ... Firm and stable, you stand among all the people and feel good ... ... They have no meaning for you ... ... You only care about your own strength ... ... which becomes stronger and stronger ... ... You look into the faces of the people passing by ... ... You feel how restless they are and feel your own calm and strength ... ... Everything is much easier when you stand upright with strong legs ... ... with strong arms and broad shoulders ... ... with your head held high ... ... just like now ... ... just like now ... ... It's easy for you to stand among people and even look them in the face ... ... Every time you look someone in the face, you feel the strength in your legs ... ... Every time you look someone in the face, you feel the strength in your arms ... ... Every time you look someone in the face, you feel the strength in your shoulders ... ... Every time you look someone in the face, you feel your head held high ... ... Every time you look someone in the face, you feel your firm gaze ... ... You want more ... ... You want to become even stronger ... ... You want to look people in the eyes and feel good about it ... ... You want to feel free ... You want to feel strong ... ... just like now ... ... So you try it out ... ... You look directly into the eyes of some who pass by and let them move on ... ... You feel strong and stable ... ... Your legs support you ... ... They are firm and strong ... ... Your arms remain strong ... ... Your shoulders are broad and become even broader and stronger ... ... Your head is straight, and your gaze is firm ... ... With every person you look in the eye, your gaze becomes firmer and stronger and you feel good ... ... With every breath, you feel freer and lighter ... ... You look into the eyes of the people passing by and feel free ... ... They move on and everything is fine ... ... You feel free and strong because you have achieved this ... ... You can do it and you feel freer and freer ... ... You want more ... ... A person stops ... ... a stranger ... ... You feel free and strong ... ... You walk up to this person and look them in the eyes ... ... You feel strong and stronger ... ... Your gaze is firm ... ... You look this person directly in the eyes and feel your own strength ... ... The deeper you look into their eyes, the stronger your power becomes ... ... The deeper you look into their eyes, the freer you feel ... ... You succeed right away ... ... You look this stranger deep in the eyes and feel your own courage ... ... You feel your strength ... ... You feel free ... ...

Just like now, it can always be ... ... You look people in the face and feel the strength in your legs and arms ... ... in your shoulders and head ... ... You look people in the face and feel courage and strength ... ... You feel liberated and can breathe deeply ... ... You can breathe freely ... ... free and calm ... ... free and calm ... ...

#2

You have a desire ... ... You want to find and strengthen the feeling of self-confidence within you ... ... You want to feel greater self-confidence than ever before ... ... and this desire becomes your goal today ... ... the most important goal of your life ... ... to finally meet people with a good feeling again ... ... Deep within you, there is every feeling in the world, including precisely this feeling of self-confidence ... ... deep inside you are strong enough and more ... ... deep inside you lies the power to achieve everything you want ... ... So you align your thoughts completely with this goal, focusing even more today on exactly what you want ... ... Self-confidence ... ... a strong self-confidence ... ... It's really amazing how much of this power is already deep within you ... ... more than you ever need ... ... because everything you can think of is already within you ... ... Today is about finding this power, and you are already succeeding today ... ... You succeed today and then every day of your life ... ...

... ... Breathe calmly and evenly into your inner center ... ... it's very simple ... ... Focus on your gut feeling and breathe deeply into your belly ... ... This sets your body to focus your strength ... ... to gather your strength and energy in your inner center ... ... You can reach your inner center by focusing on your belly ... ... because this focuses your perception, and that is what matters ... ... At the same time, your deep inner self focuses on the self-confidence lying deep within you ... ... The more you succeed in focusing your perception on your belly, the more your deep inner self succeeds in focusing on your self-confidence and awakening it for you ... ... With each breath into your belly, your self-confidence grows because more and more of your own strength and energy awakens ... ... Breathe consciously into your belly and thereby strengthen your self-confidence ... ... It's amazing how well you succeed in directing your attention inward now ... ... you are increasingly able to turn your attention inward ... ... Your gaze turns inward ... ... You feel inside yourself ... ... feel your body sensation ... ... feel your mood more and more clearly ... ... and if you think your inner mood should get better or simply change, it changes at that very moment as you want it to ... ... Your gaze turns more and more inward ... ... so far that you sink completely into your own feeling, coming closer and closer to your deeply resting self-confidence ... ... with every moment you come closer ... ... with every breath, you approach your own self-confidence, which lies deep within you waiting for you ... ... Your own self-confidence waits to be freed by you ... ... Your own strength waits to be liberated ... ... Your own courage waits to be unleashed by you ... ... today already ... ... because today is a special day ... ... today is the day of inner liberation ... ... Today is the day of self-confidence ... ... Today is your day ... ... your special day ... ... You approach the center of your strength ... ... You approach the center of your deep-seated self-confidence ... ... and reach it now ... ... You arrive now at your inner center ... ... at the center of the deep power within you ... ... Isn't it amazing how relaxed you are now? ... ... Isn't it quite remarkable that you are so calm and composed? ... ... And right now is the special moment ... ... Now it's time to really use your own power ... ...

... ... Now it's possible ... ... Now you can finally use your own power ... ... now you can finally awaken your own self-confidence ... ... it is within you ... ... It has always been within you ... ... You now awaken your self-confidence like a sleeping dog ... ... and deep within you, a light begins to shine ... ... a light of your own power and strength ... ... a light of your own courage ... ... a light of your self-confidence ... ... and this light becomes brighter and brighter with every breath ... ... You see it shining in your inner center ... ... with every breath, the light becomes brighter and your self-confidence grows ... ... with every breath, the light becomes brighter and your strength stronger ... ... with every breath, the light becomes brighter and your courage greater ... ... with every breath, the light becomes brighter and your self-assurance clearer ... ...

... ... So you let the inner light become brighter and brighter ... ... The brighter you can imagine the light within you, the greater now becomes the feeling of self-assurance, of self-confidence ... ... You let the light become even brighter ... ... The brighter you can imagine the light within you, the greater now becomes the feeling of self-assurance, of self-confidence ... ... Good ... ... very, very good ... ... It's truly amazing how easy it is for you now to let your inner light shine and become stronger ... ... really amazing how strong your self-confidence becomes as you do so ... ... You succeed ... ... You actually succeed ... ... Maybe you're already wondering how great your self-confidence will be in the end ... ... how much of it you can awaken today already ... ... when you will have succeeded in accessing your entire power and strength ... ... having the greatest courage fully at your disposal ... ... even more than today already ... ... even more than today already ... ... Let the light become even brighter because it can become even brighter ... ... much brighter ... ... The brighter you can imagine the light within you, the greater now becomes the feeling of self-assurance, of self-confidence ... ... Enjoy the moment and trust that your organism can always do this just as well as today ... ... even better from day to day ... ... because every day it becomes more natural to find your own strength ... ... you find it faster and faster every day ... ... and again and again ... ...

Your organism now prepares to always do the same ... ... Whenever you want to awaken your inner strength and make your self-confidence stronger, you consciously focus on your belly and take a deliberate breath into your belly ... ... This is the signal for your organism to immediately awaken the deep strength and courage and provide the greatest possible self-confidence … … It's very simple, even easier than today … … Whenever you consciously and deliberately breathe into your belly, your organism immediately provides you with the greatest possible self-confidence, and you feel it instantly … … Whenever you consciously and deliberately breathe into your belly, your organism immediately provides you with the greatest possible self-confidence, and you feel it instantly … …

#3

The following hypnosis session works with a physical anchor. An anchor is a trigger that is meant to evoke a specific feeling or thought. We want to help the client strengthen their feeling of self-confidence with a light pressure on the left hand (on the ball below the thumb). We discuss this with the client before the session and show them the spot they should press. During the hypnosis session, we then set the anchor. It is important to connect the pressing on the thumb ball with the already prevailing feeling of self-confidence in a state of calm. The client must feel absolutely self-confident during this session. This must be absolutely certain, otherwise, it will not work. In case of doubt, ask if they feel self-confident before setting the anchor.

You want to finally be free ... ... want to talk to other people easily and calmly ... ... This goal is your goal, and you have already done a lot for it ... ... Today you can take another big and decisive step ... ... You can set your deep inner self to feel really secure and strong ... ... free from fear and insecurity ... ... You remember that you were not always insecure ... ... there was a time in your life when you were still calm and even self-confident in dealing with people ... ... At some point, this changed, but today you turn this change back ... ... Today you become strong and courageous again, simply self-confident ... ... just like before ... ... exactly like before ... ...

... ... Today we are working with an anchor, which we have already talked about ... ... You already carry this anchor on your body ... ... your left hand is the anchor triggered by the right hand ... ... But we will come to that a little later ... ... To make full use of the anchor, find the best position to trigger it now ... ... Reach with your right hand to your left and feel for the ball of the thumb with your fingers ... ... very lightly ... ... very gently ... ... Decide whether you want to grasp it with your thumb and index finger or with your thumb and middle finger ... ... maybe you even have another way ... ... Do it in the way you can best grasp the ball of your thumb ... ... [Wait until the client has found a good grip; prompt again if they do not immediately follow] ... ... Wonderful ... ... This works best ... ... very good ... ...

And now let go of your hand again and place both hands loosely next to your body ... ...

... ... Now it's time to rediscover your old strength and calmness ... ... to revive your former self-confidence and make it even stronger than before ... ... To do this, you now go back in time ... ... You go back to a time when you were still self-confident ... ... You remember this time exactly, maybe it wasn't that long ago ... ... maybe it was years ago that you now go back ... ... Go back now to a time when you felt strongest in your life ... ... Let the images of that time come to life again ... ... Immerse yourself in this time when you were at your strongest ... ... There was this time because you were self-confident and strong before ... ... And the more you think about the strong time back then, the more you also feel this sense of security from back then ... ... The more you can now imagine how it was back then, the better you feel that this memory of strength and self-confidence exists within you ... ... You feel it now ... ... deep within you ... ... now ... ... You make it clear to yourself at this moment that you have already made a decision ... ... You have decided to be self-confident again and look ahead ... ... to shape the present and move forward into the future

... ... to take good care of yourself ... ... So you don't need more than a single second to act according to your decision ... ... From now on, you simply do what is necessary to make your decision a reality ... ... to feel that you are actually strong and self-confident as soon as you want it ... ... just like now ... ... Now, at this very moment, you can feel that this self-confidence is still within you ... ... You feel the deep desire within you to feel this feeling again and again ... ...

... ... You have decided, so you can act ... ... In the word 'act' is the word 'hand' ... ... Now you can indeed act ... ... Reach for your left hand as soon as you feel really strong inside ... ...

... ... [Wait. Give the client time. Possibly prompt again after 30 seconds or ask if they feel strong. If not, please deepen the relaxation further and promote the feeling of courage with suggestions before setting the anchor.] ... ...

... ... Do it now as you have practiced ... ... Grasp your left hand and focus on your inner feeling of self-confidence because back then you were strong ... ... If you think the feeling of strength and self-confidence should become even clearer, then let it simply become even clearer and more distinct in your feeling ... ... even more intense ... ... with even more mindfulness and care for yourself ... ... just like that ... ... just like that ... ... You can do it ... ...

... ... And now let this feeling become very conscious ... ... and now press the ball of your left hand ... ... and again ... ... press ... ... Your inner self prepares for the fact that precisely this pressing of the thumb ball is the signal to immediately feel that you are indeed self-confident and brave ... ... Whenever you press your thumb ball, you feel strong and brave and focus entirely on your feeling of self-confidence ... ... Your body is relaxed and your hands are also completely calm ... ... Your body has understood how your anchor works ... ... It has already stored it for you so that you can use it again and again ... ...

... ... Whenever you press your thumb ball, you are really strong and brave and clearly feel your own self-confidence, which becomes bigger with each press ... ... bigger with each press ... ... So it will soon become natural for you to press or massage your thumb ball again and again; it works exactly like this ... ... just like now ... ... You have decided ... ... You have acted ... ... You now return to the present and bring your own strength as a souvenir from the past to feel it every day ... ... to feel self-confidence every day of your life ... ... just like now ... ... just like now ... ...

#4

The following variation of a hypnosis session works with an anchor in the form of a handy card with the inscription "Calm and Security". An anchor is a trigger meant to evoke a specific feeling or thought. We want to help the client adjust more quickly to letting go of emerging fear in situations where they are the center of attention using a "reminder card". We discuss this with the client before the session and prepare the reminder card. It can be a labeled business card or something similar. The card is prepared and given to the client. They can hold it loosely in their hand during hypnosis or place it on their body, for example, on the solar plexus. The card should be carried with them after hypnosis, in their pocket or jacket.

You prefer to stand on the edge rather than in the center, not liking to be watched by others ... ... because you often have this feeling of insecurity and fear ... ... You intend to finally consign this fear to the past ... ... to send it to the place of memory and leave it there ... ... because that is where the past belongs ... ... only there does the past belong ... ... and every experience of fear in contact with other people is already in the past ... ... Now you are here and you are without fear ... ... You know your way around here and feel safe ... ... That's how you feel in your familiar surroundings ... ... among people you know well ... ... You don't have the fear there ... ... You can recall the experiences and past feelings of insecurity and fear in your memory, but they should not come into the present ... ... because the present belongs only to you ... ... It's important that we only hold on to the past as long as we need it to process and understand what happened ... ... You have already reached this point, that's why you are here ... ... You have processed and you have understood ... ... Therefore, now is the right time to let go ... ... to let go of the fear, to let go of the insecurity and thus to send it to the place of memory ... ...

... ... You have decided that you want to build up courage so that you can handle your daily tasks well ... ... so that you can enjoy your work and leisure time ... ... You have understood that it is you who has to turn your intentions into reality ... ... You know that it is you who makes your success

... ... and you are ready for it ... ... You are ready to give everything necessary to become inwardly calm and proud ... ... free from the old burdens of the past ... ... You have the potential for this ... ... you have the strength you need ... ...

But you want more ... ... You want to always be able to fully utilize your qualities and abilities ... ... You want to be able to quickly enter a calm state again and again ... ... especially if you should become fearful again and notice it suddenly ... ... Then you want to quickly come to a calm state that gives you security ... ...

You know the crucial words ... ... Calm and security ... ... This is the new message to yourself ... ... Calm and security ... ... This is your creed ... ... Calm and security ... ... like an inner command you give yourself ... ... Calm and security ... ... Calm and security ... ... You have a card with exactly this inscription, on your card is this goal ... ... Calm and security ... ... You feel these feelings within you now, here in a state of calm you feel calm and secure ... ... calm and secure ... ... You know you can achieve even more ... ... You can make these feelings much more intense by constantly reminding yourself of them and repeating them ... ... Calm and security ... ... The card shows it to you every day ... ... It shows you your feelings that you can recall and strengthen again and again ... ... Calm and security ... ... The card helps you become stronger every day and finally always remain calm ... ... become calm ... ... stay calm ... ... As soon as the slightest doubt arises within you, you immediately take the card in your hand and read the inscription consciously, you look at it ... ... Calm and security ... ... Then you immediately feel the effect, you feel that this is your new reality ... ... Calm and security ... ... You do it like this every day ... ... You simply let go of the fear ... ... You simply let go of the fear ... ... You read the card ... ... Calm and security ... ... The card shows it to you every day ... It shows you your own attitude, which becomes clearer every day ... ... It helps you through difficult moments ... ... As soon as the slightest doubt arises within you, you immediately take the card in your hand and look at it ... ... Calm and security ... ... Then you immediately feel the effect, you feel that this is your new reality ... ...

... ... Take your reminder card consciously in your hand now ... ... The card you feel between your fingers reminds you of it ... ... it helps you let go of the fear ... ... it helps you become calm and then remain calm ... ... free and without fear, facing the future with calm and security ... ... calm and secure ... ... every day ... ...

... ... [Now prompt the client to open their eyes and read the inscription on the reminder card while in a trance. This reinforces the effect. Opening the eyes is a fractionation, but it can be done without a special announcement or counting. Anyone can open their eyes in a trance. In a stable and deep trance, it is somewhat difficult because the client is tired and sluggish. Simply stay with suggestive prompting until the eyes open and the card is read. If you prefer to introduce the fractionation with counting steps, you can certainly do that. It is not necessary.] ...

... ... Feel the reminder card consciously between your fingers and now open your eyes and look at the card ... ... open your eyes and read what it says ... ... Calm and security ... ... Calm and security ... ... Now close your eyes again and let the words you have read work deeply within you ... ... deeply within you ...

You still feel the card between your fingers ... ... You know it reminds you every day to let go of the fear and build calm and security ... ... Whenever you take the card in your hand

and read it, you immediately feel that you become inwardly freer and calmer ... ... freer and calmer ... ... Whenever you carry the card with you, you feel lighter inside ... ... Calm and security ... ... It happens automatically because your inner self knows that this card reminds you of what you did today ... ... your own liberation ...

#5

You have decided to be able to make contact with other people more easily from today and to meet others without fear ... ... You have a goal, and you know exactly what you want ... ... To look people you meet in the eyes again and stay calm ... ... That is your goal ... ... You want to be able to speak freely and calmly with strangers, especially when the attention is on you ... ... You know others can do it, and you even know people who can do it very well ... ... And you know everything is fine as soon as you can do it just like them ... ... and today is a very special day ... ... Today you can learn from a person who can be your role model ... ... You know people who could be your role models because they talk to others without fear ... ... Let images of such people come before your inner eye and choose the person who can do it best ... ... a person you would like to learn from how to be relaxed and calm in conversation, while also being self-confident and assured ... ... You know such people ... ... Sometimes you even think all people are so relaxed ... ... But now you choose the person who can do it best to learn from them in a special way today ... ... Maybe you wonder how quickly you can learn from this person to proceed just like them ... ... to be just as relaxed and confident ... ... maybe you are already thinking about how nice it will be once you have managed to act exactly like them ...

So watch your role model closely ... ... Observe this person in a situation that has often been difficult for you ... ... maybe in conversation with one person or in a group of people ... ... however you want, choose a situation ... ... This person can do it quite naturally ... ... It is the way this person approaches the situation ... ... setting themselves internally for success ... ... Like an invisible observer, you stand behind this person who has never been afraid, and watch how they do it ... ... It's truly remarkable how well this person can do everything ... ... how well they handle challenges ...

So you look through the eyes of the role model to see how good this perspective is when you can do everything you have set out to do ... ... It feels good and so simple because your role model can do it ... ... And you learn from the role model by looking through their eyes ... ... as if this person were lending you their eyes or letting you see through their eyes ... ... You see the situation entirely from the perspective of your role model ... ... and you see that it is a relaxed and yet proud look ... ... a good perspective for you too ... ... Then you go into the body feeling of the role model, as if you could slip into this person like a spirit ... ... You go into the body feeling and consciously perceive how this person moves ... ... so self-assured and strong ... ... Feel how a self-assured and strong body feels ... ... Your role model does it for you and with you in this moment ... ... It feels good ... ... It feels right, and above all, it is so natural and easy because your role model does everything for you and with you ... ... as if the strong body of the role model were your own body at this moment ... ... You feel this physical strength, and at this moment, you realize how much the body has to do with your own feeling ... ... Thus, your own posture already changes, the tension rises, and your body becomes more stable in its appearance ...

You want to learn more ... ... Then you go into the mood of your role model ... ... It's truly surprising that the inner mood is cheerful and happy ... ... Your role model even enjoys talking to or being with other people, being the center of attention ... ... being observed is interesting and exciting ... ... It feels good ... ... It feels completely normal to be in the center ... ... It feels familiar ... ... It feels ordinary ... ... because your role model can do all this and does it right now for you and with you ... ... Your own inner mood becomes just as cheerful and happy, and at this moment, together with your role model, you feel just as comfortable and free in the center as this person does ... ... you succeed just as your role model does ... ... because you can here and today, in this very moment, actually adopt the characteristics of your role model ... ... Now completely replace the image of your role model with your own ... ... Step entirely into the world of your role model, whoever it is ... ... Be like this person and observe that you can act exactly like them ... ... just as self-assured ... ... just as confident ... ... just as calm ... ... You can do it because you have learned it intensely today and deeply internalized it ... ... You have understood it ... ... and even more astonishing is that all this was already within you ... ... The strength was already within you ... ... The calmness was already within you ... ... The confidence was already within you ... ... You found all this deep within you ... ... You know your role model, but you know it is your role model because this person does what is within you and has been discovered by you today ... ... strengthened today ... ... You are and remain strong and courageous ... ... You move like your role model ... ... You have the gaze and perspective of your role model ... ... You have the same good feelings as your role model ... ... You yourself are your new role model from today on ... ...

Your organism firmly imprints these good qualities of your role model so that you yourself can access them anytime ... ... Your entire inner self prepares to provide you with these good and helpful qualities of your role model whenever you meet other people or are addressed ... ... These qualities are available to you from your deep inner self especially when you are in the center of attention ... ... you succeed in being calm and staying calm ... ... just like today here ... ... just like today ... ...

#6

You know the fear of other people, which is not really fear of the people themselves but the fear that you might embarrass yourself ... ... the fear that you might stand out and then be judged badly ... ... or suddenly lose control ... ... You fear that you might not be able to speak or only very shakily ... ... you probably have experienced something like this before ... ... Then at some point, you began to feel this fear more and more often ... ... always being shaky and fearful in contact with people ... ... Maybe you have already wished you had a stable protection around you so that nothing could happen to you ... ... so that you are shielded and protected ... ... like a safety zone directly around your body ... ... so stable that no one can get too close to you ... ... so that no judgments or opinions can come too close ... ... so that much bounces off you or better yet, bounces off before it even reaches you ... ... a protective dome would surely be helpful ... ... a glass dome from which you can look out, where you can be seen and perceived, but you are simply safe ... ... and precisely this idea can help you more easily connect with people ... ... to feel more secure ... ... because all the thoughts and images in your head also produce feelings ... ... and if you have the image of a glass protective dome around you in your head, as an idea, then you also feel much safer ... ... Maybe you are surprised that such a simple trick can actually work ... ... It can work and it will work ... ...

... ... Now imagine there is exactly this protective dome around your body ... ... Imagine, deep in your inner images and thus automatically in your feelings, that a protective dome surrounds your body ... ... and at the same time, pay attention to the feeling within you ... ... now you are relaxed and can feel comfortable ... ... really relaxed and you can feel really comfortable ... ... Imagine how you could move in your everyday life with this protective dome ... ... Imagine the protective dome cannot be penetrated by anyone, and if you want, others cannot even see into it ... ... It is an idea ... ... it is an inner image ... ... it is a fantasy, but fantasy and reality are very close together ... ... What you can imagine also arises in your feelings at the same time ... ... So imagine exactly how it would be if you had this protective dome around you ... ... At the same time, the feeling of being protected arises within you ... ... maybe you already feel it a bit more clearly ... ... maybe you will feel it even more clearly in a few moments or in a few minutes ... ... You are protected because there is this protective dome ... ... It is within you ... ... You protect yourself with this image ... ... It works ... ... It works now in your imagination and then also in your waking reality, because it all depends on your thoughts ... ... Your thoughts could produce fear, and often you thought about what bad or embarrassing things could happen ... ... Now you imagine something different ... ... You imagine the protective dome ... ... and again your body reacts to it ... ... and again your whole organism reacts to it ... ... with the feeling of actually being protected, and you are ... ... protected by inner images and by the feeling of security ... ... The image of the protective dome is connected at this moment firmly and inseparably with the feeling of security ... ... even more firmly ... ... The image of the protective dome is connected at this moment firmly and inseparably with the feeling of security ... ... It works ... ... It works now in your imagination and then also in your waking reality, because it all depends on your thoughts ... ... It all depends now on this one thought ... ... on this one image of the protective dome around your body ... ... You see the protective dome before your inner eye ... ... You see the protective dome in your inner images ... ... You feel this protective dome around your body in your imagination ... ... You imagine the protective dome as clearly as you can ... ... The more you focus on this image of a protective dome, the more intense the feeling of security becomes, inseparably connected with it ... ... So imagine the protective dome around your body even more clearly ... ... Observe yourself in your everyday life and imagine that this protective dome surrounds your body ... ... good ... ... The more you focus on this image of a protective dome, the more intense the feeling of security becomes, inseparably connected with it ... ... It works now in your imagination and then also in your waking reality, because it all depends on your thoughts ... ... Your thoughts could produce fear, and often you thought about what bad or embarrassing things could happen ... ... Now your thoughts produce the feeling of security ... ... now and again ... ... now and again ...

You firmly imprint this ... ... Thoughts produce feelings ... ... Thoughts produce feelings ... ... That's how fear arose ... ... That's how the feeling of security arises now ... ... now in a state of relaxation ... ... and every day when you imagine your protective dome ... ... and as soon as you leave your home, you imagine your protective dome every day ... ... You put it on when you go outside and then you immediately feel the feeling of security because both are firmly connected ... ... the image of the protective dome and the feeling of security ... ... As soon as you imagine the dome, the feeling of security automatically arises ... ... Only this is possible ... ... Protective dome and security ... ... Protective dome and security ... ... Only this is possible ...

#7

Ideomotorics refers to the phenomenon that our body follows our feelings and thoughts with movements. In everyday life, this following is shown as posture, muscle tension, and movement patterns of a person, which naturally change with mood and thoughts. In trance, ideomotoric signals can be used to obtain information that the client cannot actively communicate. For example, the subconscious can answer questions with an agreed-upon finger signal. Of course, ideomotoric reactions can also be used suggestively, for example, in arm levitations and catalepsies.

The following application can be done without a trance induction and is therefore all the more impactful. An ideomotoric reaction (upward movement of the right arm and downward movement of the left arm) is created to show the client that it is the images and ideas in their thoughts that create their truth of social phobia. This is meant to strengthen the belief in the possibility of change through new thoughts and new images. Of course, the whole thing can also be done after a detailed trance induction, but I recommend foregoing this because it leaves more of an impression. Experienced hypnotists know: Ideomotorics work without hypnosis, but if it works, it is hypnosis!

You probably can't simply read the following text like the others. I still want to encourage you to try this variant once. It's not about the wording but the approach. You don't need to learn every word by heart.

Explain to your client now that they should stand and stretch both arms forward. The palm of the left hand should face up, and the palm of the right hand should face down. Then they should imagine that a heavy object, a thick book, or a stone lies on the left hand. At the same time, they should imagine that a gas-filled balloon is tied to the right wrist with a string. Then suggest that the heavy object pushes the left hand down and the gas balloon pulls the right hand up. Repeat the suggestion several times. Very quickly, the left arm will move down, and the right arm will move up. The client simultaneously feels that the left arm actually gets heavier and the right one lighter. This is a simple exercise that is sometimes done as a suggestibility test. It always works, even if a client tries to resist the effect. They feel it, and their arms will visibly react to it. The whole thing can happen with a very wide scissor movement of the arms or with "only" ten centimeters distance. But that is enough. Clients are impressed by the exercise even if they already know it. And it still works then. Just try it yourself without suggestion: What happens when you stretch your arms forward as described and imagine both images, heavy stone, and gas balloon, with your eyes closed?

You will see: Your arms will react to it!

Of course, you don't need a text template because you don't need to read this simple exercise. Still, I have written a short text example here as orientation. I often do the exercise in courses and prefer to work standing. But it also works sitting or lying on a narrow couch.

Text Instruction as Orientation:

... ... Stand up straight, stable on both legs. And now stretch your arms forward. Very loosely, do not overextend. Good. Now turn the palm of your left hand up so that you could place something on it. And the right hand faces down. Good, it's starting ... ...

… … Close your eyes and keep your arms like this … … Now imagine placing a very heavy stone on your left hand … … In your imagination, place a heavy stone on your left hand, and at the right wrist, tie a gas-filled balloon … …

… … On the left hand lies a very heavy stone, and the right hand is pulled up by the balloon … …

… … On the left hand lies a very heavy stone, and the right hand is pulled up by the balloon … …

[Repeat the two images and observe the client's arms. You don't need a special trance tone in your voice. You can keep talking "normally," maybe even a bit faster than usual. Repeat the two images either always the same or with other words until the left arm slowly moves down and the right one moves up. This will happen very quickly. It's very simple and succeeds with everyone, even laypeople without trance and without any knowledge of hypnosis, trance, or suggestion.]

… … Now keep your arms like this and open your eyes now … … Look at your arms! … …

Let the client marvel now. Most people are very surprised that it worked. The movement of the arms is usually felt even with closed eyes, but many are unsure if it is a trick, whether they just imagined the movement. The more intense is the surprise that the arms have actually and (usually) moved so far. Discuss again with the client that it is only the images in their head that create this reality. Similarly, it is only the images in their head that produce their fear. Conversely, this of course means that new images or new thoughts can also produce new attitudes.

This exercise is quite boring as a suggestibility test because nobody needs such a test. As an introduction to therapy, however, the exercise can be very appropriate and helpful to show, for example, that images and ideas can actually influence us very quickly and clearly, against the knowledge of our mind. The mind knows that there is no object on the left hand and no balloon pulling on the right. Suggest to the client to repeat the exercise again to see and check for themselves that the effect is also noticeable when they know beforehand what will happen.

#8

You know this difficulty in making contact with others ... ... often having the feeling of not being seen or being rejected ... ... then you developed fear that became stronger and stronger ... ... You have wondered where this fear comes from and why you could not let it go in the past ... ... and today you are here to finally do just that ... ... to let go of your fear and then naturally encounter other people again ... ... to be able to meet strangers with a relaxed feeling and look forward with curiosity to what you may experience with them ... ... Maybe you know that everything in our feelings is also in our body ... ... Your body reacts to every feeling, to the beautiful feelings as well as to fear ... ... and your body can also signal to you what feeling you can have ... ... Because feelings change posture ... ... and posture, in turn, influences the feeling ... ... When fear comes, everything feels tight, you can't breathe properly ... ... when you feel secure, you can breathe deeply ... ... and when you feel really free, you can breathe in deeply and exhale vigorously ... ... your chest expands with your breath, and you also feel this free feeling in your body ... ... So, conversely, breathing can help you feel freer and more secure ... ... because whenever you might feel insecure, even if only the slightest fear arises, you can help yourself become free and secure by breathing deeply and openly ... ... You can train your body today to do this for you ... ... To do this, you continue to relax ... ... You relax deeper and deeper ... ... let yourself drift in comfort ... ... Here everything is fine ... ... Here you are completely safe ... ... Here you can rest without any fear ... ... You feel good ... ... You can already focus on your breathing and continue to breathe calmly ... ... calmly let your breath flow ... ... Simply feel your calm breathing rhythm ... ... The more you focus on the flow of your breath, the deeper you relax ... ... by itself ... ... Pay attention to the flow of your breath and allow yourself to relax ... ... simply sink deeper and deeper into a beautiful relaxation ... ... deeper and deeper ... ... just like that ... ... just like that ... ... At this moment, you can feel completely free and secure ... ... completely free and secure because there is nothing to do here ... ... You feel free and secure ... ... completely free and secure ... ... and your body feels it too ... ... You can make this feeling of freedom and security even more intense

...... Breathe deeply now and feel your chest expand ...... [Wait for a deep breath] ...... good ...... once more ...... [Wait for a deep breath] ...... You're doing it just right ......

...... Feel how your chest expands with deep breathing because that makes the feeling of freedom even stronger ...... the feeling of security even more intense ...... Continue breathing with deep breaths ...... and focus on this feeling of opening and expanding ...... of freedom ...... [Wait for a deep breath] ...... good ...... [Wait for a deep breath] ...... You're doing it just right ...... It's working ...... It's working right now ...... The more you focus on the feeling in your body and feel the movement of your lungs expanding, the more your body succeeds in expanding this feeling of freedom ...... Your body learns for you to breathe deeply whenever fear could arise, to strengthen the feeling of freedom just like now ...... The fear becomes smaller, and you let it go with the exhale ......

You continue to train your body ...... Breathe deeply and feel the freedom ...... [Wait for the inhale, then immediately continue reading] ...... Exhale slowly and long and let go of the rest of the fear ...... [Wait for the exhale, then immediately continue reading] ...... Continue breathing calmly ... ... very calmly and feel the pleasant feeling of freedom and security ... ... good ... ... and once more ... ... Breathe deeply and feel the freedom ... ... [Wait for the inhale, then immediately continue reading] ... ... Exhale slowly and long and let go of the rest of the fear ... ... [Wait for the exhale, then immediately continue reading] ... ... Continue breathing calmly ... ... very calmly and feel the pleasant feeling of freedom and security ... ... good ... ... You can do it ... ... Your body learns with each breath to make the feeling of freedom and security stronger and let go of the rest of the fear until it is completely gone ... ... until even the last bit of fear is gone ... ... and once more ... ... Breathe deeply and feel the freedom ... ... [Wait for the inhale, then immediately continue reading] ... ... Exhale slowly and long and let go of the rest of the fear ... ... [Wait for the exhale, then immediately continue reading] ... ... Continue breathing calmly ... ... very calmly and feel the pleasant feeling of freedom and security ... ... good ... ... Allow yourself now to rest and relax ... ... Simply enjoy the pleasant feeling of relaxation and trust that your body takes care of everything and always helps you ... ... to let go of fear and find a feeling of freedom and security ...

Your body knows how to do this and imprints everything exactly so that it can help you every day to meet people with a good and secure feeling ... ... Whenever you consciously breathe deeply in and exhale slowly and long, your body provides you with the feeling of freedom and security and at the same time lets go of the fear ... ... This works also and especially in a waking state ... ... every day of your life ... ... every single day, just like today ... ... just like today ...

#9

Somewhere in your imagination, there is a very special place … … a place where you can find refuge … … where only you decide what can be … … a land of peace and freedom … … of security and safety … … the land of your dreams … … Whatever you have lost in your life … … whatever you have missed … … what you have searched for in vain and with despair … … Here you find everything you need to live freely and happily … … Here you find everything you need to experience healing … … because here you always find yourself … … So you set off, in your thoughts and in your imagination, you start the journey … … You go to the land of dreams … …

You stand in front of a high wall covered with moss … … You walk along this wall and find an iron gate … … On the gate hangs a sign with the inscription "Garden of Time" … … You decide to enter the garden … … You open the iron gate, which opens easily and grants you entry into the Garden of Time … … You look around the garden … … You see a beautiful and well-kept garden with fragrant flowers … …

with blossoming trees and others already bearing ripe fruits ... ... There are beds that look beautifully ordered and well-kept ... ... as if a gardener were here every day to keep everything in order and create beauty ... ... the Garden of Time ... ... the garden of your time ... ... the garden of your lifetime ... ... You walk between the plants and beds and enjoy the beauty of the garden ... ... Along the way, you also find areas of the garden that look different ... ... dried up ... ... and barren ... ... with withered plants and overgrown shrubs ... ... These areas also exist in the Garden of Time ... ... but in a special way, even these spots are beautiful ... ... The whole garden seems familiar and known to you ... ... It's as if you've been here many times ... ... Then you come to an area of the garden where only very young plants grow ... ... tiny shoots just sprouting from the ground ... ... and there you find footprints ... ... small footprints ... ... the footprints of a child ... ... You follow them ... ... Then you see a child in the Garden of Time ... ... it sits between shrubs, in the shade, and holds a book in its hand ... ... You sit down next to the child, and then you realize that you know this child ... ... you've seen its face many times before ... ... long ago, many years ago ... ...

you've often heard its voice ... ... you still hear it in the wind ... ... and at night when you can't sleep ... ... You hear it softly even during the day when the fear of people comes ... ... when you become insecure and fearful in contact with other people ... ... You know the voice that sounds like your childhood voice used to ... ... Then you recognize in the child's face your own face ... ... in its voice your own voice ... ... and in its fear your own fear ... ... You recognize yourself ... ... You meet yourself in another time ... ... The child by your side ... ... your inner child ... ... opens the book it holds in its hands ... ... Then you notice that it is a photo album ... ... with pictures of the past ... ... Pictures of your childhood and your entire life ... ... You look at pictures of your childhood ... ... your first bike ... ... your favorite place ... ... Toys are there too ... ... and the people who were part of your family ... ... maybe parents ... ... maybe siblings too ... ... maybe grandparents or other people ... ... You remember your childhood ... ... back then your fear slowly began ... ... Maybe you didn't have fear back then ... ... you might even think it only really started in your adult life ... ... and yet there were events back then that contributed to your fear of people building up ... ... You see the pictures of the past ... ... They show you how it was back then ... ... and with the pictures come memories of the feelings of childhood ... ... maybe fear ... ... or loneliness ... ... maybe sadness ... ... or longing ... ... You feel once again what the child once felt ... ... You experience once again the mood of that time ... ... feel once again the emotions the child once had ... ... this feeling that is still within you today ... ... The child by your side, in the land of dreams, feels it too ... ... Your inner child feels what you feel ... ... Your inner child knows what you know ... ... Your inner child remembers what you remember ... ... Your inner child wants what you want ... ... It wants to leave all this behind ... ... to free itself from the fear of the past because it started back then ... ... The child admires and envies you because you have grown up ... ... That's exactly what the child by your side wishes for, in the land of dreams ... ... the child within you ... ... It wants to let go and be grown-up ... ... just like you ... ... exactly like you ... ... That's why you are here ... ... to put everything in order here and now ... ... and that is easier than you think ... ... Back then, the fear arose, it couldn't have happened otherwise ... ... It wasn't your fault ... ... You simply couldn't tell anyone your true feelings because no one was there ... ... or because you didn't want to burden anyone and thought you had to handle it yourself ... ... Today it is different ... ... Here and now, you feel what you feel ... ... feel the feelings of the past as they were ... ... and with that, everything changes because now you can learn anew and differently from all this, deep within you ... ... You learn quite naturally in the land of dreams how it works, to be self-confident and courageous ... ... You have always been brave, always kept going and persevered ... ... already persevering back then, even though you were so alone ... ... You have shown more courage and strength than you could see yourself ... ... You now learn deeply in the land of dreams how to feel this courage and strength every day ... ... and the child by your side learns with you ...

You close your eyes and rest ... ... You dream of yourself and the inner child ... ... dream that both of you go your way self-confidently and courageously ... ... today already ... ... or tomorrow ... ... or every day of your future life a great piece ... ... then you think about the fact that the land of dreams is deep within you ... ... It was always there ... ... I'm just telling you about it ...

#10

Somewhere in your imagination, there is a very special place ... ... a place where you can find refuge ... ... where only you decide what can be ... ... a land of peace and freedom ... ... of security and safety ... ... the land of your dreams ... ... Whatever you have lost in your life ... ... whatever you have missed ... ... what you have searched for in vain and with despair ... ... Here you find everything you need to live freely and happily ... ... Here you find everything you need to experience healing ... ... because here you always find yourself ... ... So you set off, in your thoughts and in your imagination, you start the journey ... ... You go to the land of dreams ... ...

You stand on a meadow and see three large crystal balls in front of you, so large that you can stand upright in them ... ... You walk to the left ball and look inside ... ... It is empty ... ... So you go into the ball to look at it from the inside ... ... This ball is the ball of your successes ... ... and you have had many successes in your life, more than you might have thought ... ... and slowly images arise around you, like in a cinema you see images from your childhood and stand in the middle of it ... ... As a small child, you already had successes ... ... maybe you once searched for something you missed very much ... ... then you finally found it, and that was a great success for you ... ... You were happy and proud to have it again ... ... or you once built something, assembled a puzzle or a model, and then you were happy and proud when you finished it ... ... You have always achieved and accomplished things in your life ... ... even in school, you had successes ... ... maybe many or just a few but special ones ... ... The rare success weighs all the more heavily ... ... Now you remember the seemingly small events of your life that were successes for you ... ... whether seemingly small or large successes ... ... There have been and still are successes in your life ... ... Even now, in your adult life, there have been and are successes ... ... You look at them ... ... The images come to you naturally ... ... They arise in your memory and show themselves in the ball of successes ... ... So you can feel the power of success once more and internally prepare yourself to be successful again ... ... to successfully work on being able to approach people more easily again, to meet them more easily ... ... with a good feeling ... ... with a feeling of success ... ... Then you go outside, leave the ball, and carry your own success power with you ... ... You carry it within you ... ... Then you go to the second ball, which is a ball of overcoming ... ... You have already overcome so much ... ... overcome boundaries ... ... You see memories and images from your life again ... ... Maybe you remember climbing a closet as a small child or over a high wall ... ... maybe the wall wasn't so high from today's perspective, but from the eyes and body of the child, it was still a difficult boundary that you overcame ... ... Maybe you once achieved something in school that you thought was beyond your possibilities ... ... Even then, you had overcome a boundary ... ... Again and again, you were faced with the challenge of achieving more than you thought you were capable of ... ... Even living with the fear and continuing was a great challenge you repeatedly took on ... ... It cost a lot of strength, but you faced it again and again, always overcoming boundaries ... ... always overcoming your own boundaries ... ... That is what you need now again ... ... you need your own ability to overcome boundaries again to now overcome the boundaries of fear and let it go ... ... You take your own power of overcoming ... ... It shows itself to you once more in images of your memory ... ... You have this power, and you use it to overcome the boundaries of fear ... ... You leave the ball and carry the power of overcoming within you ... ... It helps you to let go of your fear and be self-confident and strong again ... ... You go to the third ball, which is a ball of letting go ... ... You enter the ball again, and the images start playing like in a movie ... ... You have had to let go of so much in your life ... ... even as a child, you had to let go ... ... Maybe you lost something, a beloved object or a beloved person you had to let go of ... ... in school, friendships formed and also passed, you had to let go there too ... ... Even in your adult life, you often had to let go ... ... and sometimes you were the one who liked to let go ... ... because you were better off letting go ... ... because you felt freer after letting go of an idea ... ... after letting go of a person ... ... You see the images of your memory once more ... ... You had to let go ... ... You often wanted to let go ... ... You could always let go and thus became free for new things ... ... You can use that again now ... ... can use your own ability to let go to finally let go of the fear or let go of it again and again ... ... You perceive this ability within you again ... ... You leave the ball and carry the ability to let go within you ... ...

... ... Then you find a nice spot on the meadow and lie down ... ... You close your eyes and start dreaming ... ... You dream a beautiful dream of a time when you have no more fear at all and feel really comfortable in contact and dealing with other people ... ... really comfortable ...

You think about how quickly you will succeed in letting go of the fear completely and meeting other people freely and relaxed again ... ... You consider that this might happen today already or at least a large part of it today ... ... and then a bit more each day in your life until you have completely achieved it ... ... being successful and letting go ... ... overcoming boundaries again ... ... Then you think about the fact that the land of dreams is deep within you ... ... It was always there ... ... I'm just telling you about it ...

Distribution, publication, and copying in any form are prohibited and subject to damages.

Overview of All Titles in the Series "Ten Hypnoses"

Volume 1: Smoking Cessation
Volume 2: Anxiety and Restlessness
Volume 3: Burnout
Volume 4: Reducing Overweight
Volume 5: Coping with the Past
Volume 6: Suicidal Thoughts and Attempts
Volume 7: Psycho-Oncology
Volume 8: Obsessions and Tics
Volume 9: Self-Confidence and Decision-Making
Volume 10: Grief Work
Volume 11: Psychosomatics
Volume 12: Chronic Pain
Volume 13: Depressive Thoughts
Volume 14: Panic Attacks
Volume 15: Domestic Violence, Victim Support
Volume 16: Post-Traumatic Stress
Volume 17: Exam Anxiety and Stage Fright
Volume 18: Anti-Violence Training, Offender Support
Volume 19: Addiction Tendencies
Volume 20: Social Phobia and Fear of Contact
Volume 21: Nail Biting
Volume 22: Self-Awareness and Self-Love
Volume 23: Teeth Grinding and Night Clenching
Volume 24: Feelings of Guilt
Volume 25: Fear in Crowds
Volume 26: Fear of Flying, Aviophobia
Volume 27: Fear in Enclosed Spaces, Claustrophobia
Volume 28: Tinnitus, Ear Noises
Volume 29: Fear of Heights
Volume 30: Neurodermatitis

Copying, publishing, and sharing with third parties are only permitted with the written consent of the author. Please observe the notes on copyright and usage.

Volume 31: Finding Inner Balance
Volume 32: Overcoming Loneliness
Volume 33: Fear of Illness, Hypochondria
Volume 34: Anticipatory Anxiety, Fear of Fear
Volume 35: Jealousy in Relationships
Volume 36: Driving Anxiety
Volume 37: New Start after Separation
Volume 38: Fear of Injections
Volume 39: Heart Anxiety Neurosis
Volume 40: Overcoming Resentment and Anger
Volume 41: Resolving Blockages and Positive Thinking
Volume 42: Stress Reduction, Stress Management
Volume 43: Body Relaxation
Volume 44: Deep Relaxation
Volume 45: Fear of the Dark
Volume 46: Falling Asleep and Staying Asleep
Volume 47: Compulsive Buying
Volume 48: Restless Legs Syndrome
Volume 49: Bulimia
Volume 50: Anorexia
Volume 51: Overcoming Nightmares
Volume 52: Imagined Deformity
Volume 53: Overcoming Distrust, Finding Trust
Volume 54: Processing Failures
Volume 55: Humiliation, Emotional Hurt
Volume 56: Distressing Compassion, Vicarious Suffering
Volume 57: Self-Forgiveness
Volume 58: Self-Awareness, Self-Confidence
Volume 59: Saying No
Volume 60: Assertiveness
Volume 61: Setting Boundaries and Self-Assertion
Volume 62: Decision-Making Ability

Volume 63: Success Orientation
Volume 64: Ruminating, Circular Thinking
Volume 65: Accepting Pregnancy
Volume 66: Birth Preparation
Volume 67: Spiritual Opening
Volume 68: Joy of Life and Inner Lightness
Volume 69: Patience and Inner Peace
Volume 70: Fibromyalgia and Rheumatism
Volume 71: Irritable Bowel Syndrome, Crohn's Disease
Volume 72: Fear of Nausea, Emetophobia
Volume 73: Stuttering and Cluttering, Speech Flow Disorders
Volume 74: Concentration and Knowledge Anchoring
Volume 75: Vitality and Spontaneity
Volume 76: Searching for Meaning and Finding Goals
Volume 77: Life Crises, Life Events
Volume 78: Workaholism, Goal Obsession
Volume 79: Helper Syndrome, Helpless Helpers
Volume 80: Medication Abuse
Volume 81: Gambling Addiction
Volume 82: Internet Addiction, Smartphone Addiction
Volume 83: Hoarding Disorder, Compulsive Collecting
Volume 84: Conspiracy Thoughts, Overvalued Ideas
Volume 85: Fear of Operations and Treatments
Volume 86: Fear of Aging
Volume 87: Travel Anxiety
Volume 88: Anxiety When Urinating, Paruresis
Volume 89: Fear of Intimacy and Togetherness
Volume 90: Fear of Blushing
Volume 91: Coming Out in Homosexuality
Volume 92: Charisma Training
Volume 93: Migraines and Chronic Headaches
Volume 94: Overcoming Allergies, Bronchial Asthma

Volume 95: Normalizing Blood Pressure
Volume 96: Compulsive Perfectionism
Volume 97: Sports Hypnosis, Motivation
Volume 98: Sports Hypnosis, Performance Enhancement
Volume 99: Determination and Focus
Volume 100: Encountering the Inner Child
Volume 101: Cravings, Binge Eating
Volume 102: Stimulating Metabolism
Volume 103: Bipolar Mood Swings
Volume 104: Borderline, Identity Crises
Volume 105: Hypomania, Euphoria, Mania
Volume 106: Restlessness, Agitation
Volume 107: Nervous Breakdown
Volume 108: Adjustment Disorders
Volume 109: Self-Alienation, Depersonalization
Volume 110: Ending Self-Pity
Volume 111: Primary Gain of Illness
Volume 112: Secondary Gain of Illness
Volume 113: Bullying, Victim Support
Volume 114: Letting Go of Envy and Jealousy
Volume 115: Fear of Spiders, Arachnophobia
Volume 116: Fear of Dogs or Cats
Volume 117: Fear of Strangers, Xenophobia
Volume 118: Excessive Worries, Generalized Anxiety
Volume 119: Strengthening Sense of Responsibility
Volume 120: Unrequited Love, Heartache
Volume 121: Work-Life Balance
Volume 122: Letting Go of Unattainable Goals
Volume 123: Allowing and Accepting Help
Volume 124: Letting Go of Adult Children
Volume 125: Tourette Syndrome
Volume 126: Life Changes and New Starts

Volume 127: Accepting Life in a Wheelchair
Volume 128: Understanding and Overcoming Homesickness
Volume 129: Understanding and Overcoming Wanderlust
Volume 130: Dizziness, Meniere's Disease
Volume 131: Overcoming Aggression
Volume 132: Cutting and Self-Harm
Volume 133: Hair Pulling, Trichotillomania
Volume 134: Postpartum Depression
Volume 135: For Relatives of Dementia Patients
Volume 136: Self-Harm, Artificial Disorders
Volume 137: Activating Self-Healing Powers
Volume 138: Preventing Depression Relapse
Volume 139: Reactive Psychoses, Follow-Up
Volume 140: Obsessive Thoughts and Impulses
Volume 141: Compulsive Checking
Volume 142: Compulsive Counting, Symmetry Obsession
Volume 143: Compulsive Washing, Cleanliness Obsession
Volume 144: Compulsive Questioning
Volume 145: Dissociative Paralysis
Volume 146: Phantom Pain
Volume 147: Overcoming Complaining
Volume 148: Hay Fever, Pollen Allergy
Volume 149: Sexual Abuse, Victim Support
Volume 150: Standing Strong Against Sexism, #metoo
Volume 151: Binge Eating
Volume 152: Overcoming Thoughts of Revenge
Volume 153: Detachment from the Aggressor, Stockholm Syndrome
Volume 154: Courage to Separate
Volume 155: Chronic Fatigue, Exhaustion
Volume 156: Fear of the Future, Existential Anxiety
Volume 157: Excessive Worry About Children
Volume 158: Fear of Failure

Volume 159: Ending Distrust and Control
Volume 160: Dejection, Dysphoria
Volume 161: Boreout, Chronic Boredom
Volume 162: Bipolar Disorders, Relapse Prevention
Volume 163: Mania, Relapse Prevention
Volume 164: Nihilism, Feelings of Worthlessness
Volume 165: Thumb Sucking
Volume 166: Being Brave
Volume 167: Being Proud
Volume 168: Overcoming Shyness
Volume 169: Being Able to Delegate Responsibility
Volume 170: Being Able to Show Emotions
Volume 171: Letting Go of Guilt, Victim Support
Volume 172: Processing Guilt, Offender Support
Volume 173: Mood Swings, Cyclothymia
Volume 174: Lack of Drive, Vital Sadness
Volume 175: Hearing Voices with Reality Reference
Volume 176: Confident Communication
Volume 177: Standing Up for Oneself
Volume 178: Taking New Paths
Volume 179: Confident Job Application
Volume 180: No Longer Being Taken Advantage Of
Volume 181: End of Submissiveness
Volume 182: Depressive Numbness
Volume 183: Mood Drops, Affective Incontinence
Volume 184: Mood Instability
Volume 185: Somatoform Disorders
Volume 186: Stomach Ulcer, Psychosomatic
Volume 187: Accepting Amputation
Volume 188: Overcoming and Letting Go of Hatred
Volume 189: Ending Accusations
Volume 190: Allowing Tears, Being Able to Cry

Volume 191: Finding and Sorting Repressed Feelings
Volume 192: Somatoform Pain
Volume 193: Living Autonomously
Volume 194: Anhedonia, Joylessness
Volume 195: Persistent Sadness
Volume 196: Obesity, Food Addiction
Volume 197: Parents of Abused Children
Volume 198: Letting Go and Letting Be
Volume 199: Childhood Sexual Abuse
Volume 200: Fear of Loss

www.ingramcontent.com/pod-product-compliance
Lightning Source LLC
Chambersburg PA
CBHW030459220526
45464CB00006B/2578